Battling Gout Cookbook

Brilliant Gout Recipes for A Hectic Lifestyle

BY

Stephanie Sharp

Copyright © 2019 by Stephanie Sharp

WWWWWWWWWWWWWWWWWWWWWWWWWWWWWWWWWWWWWW

License Notes

wwwwwwwwwwwwwwwwwwwwwwwwwwwwwwwwwwwwwwwww

Table of Contents

Introduction

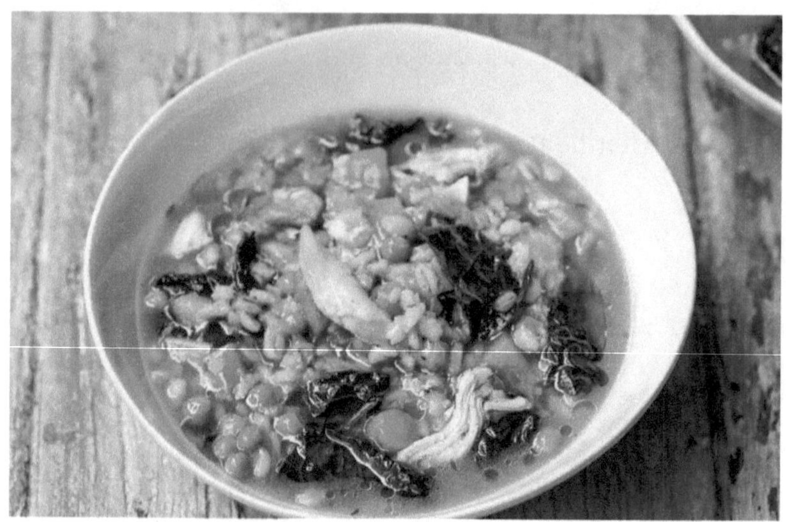

Finally, there is a relief for gout!

A proper diet is the number one way to relieve your gout pains.

Gout Cookbook is dedicated to bringing you the most effective and safest homeopathic and natural remedies that are guaranteed to work when properly applied.

We understand the health concerns of persons and some persons have had firsthand experience with this disorder. We are not miracle workers nor do we have all the answers but the ingredients used to prepare these recipes will aid in pain relief and everyone can enjoy these recipes. Even though they are specific to the relief of gout, the recipes are designed to satisfy your taste buds, easily prepared and can be enjoyed by the entire family.

Carrot Juice

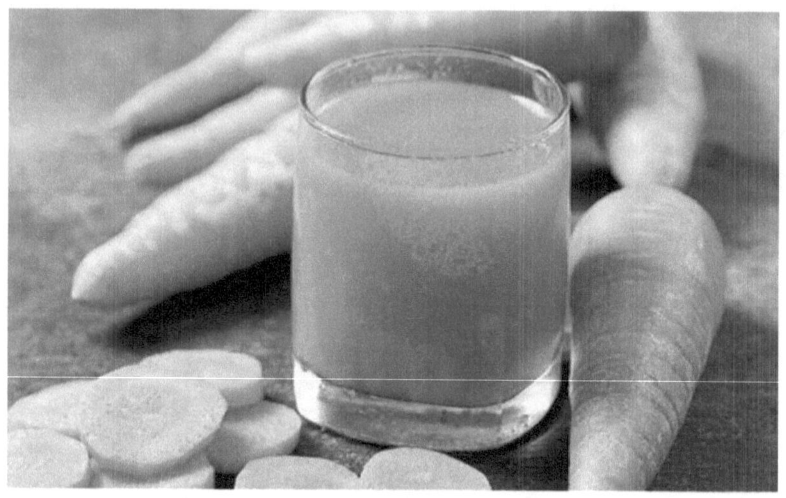

A hearty, healthy Carrot Juice. Very authentic and refreshing.

Serves: 1

Time: 15 mins.

Ingredients:

- 2 sticks of celery
- ½" ginger
- 1 carrot, large
- ½ cucumber
- 2 apples, green
- ½ lemon

Directions:

1. Add ingredients to a blender and pulse on high settings for a minute or two until smooth.

2. Transfer the mixture to a large glass. Serve & enjoy!

Licorice Root Tea

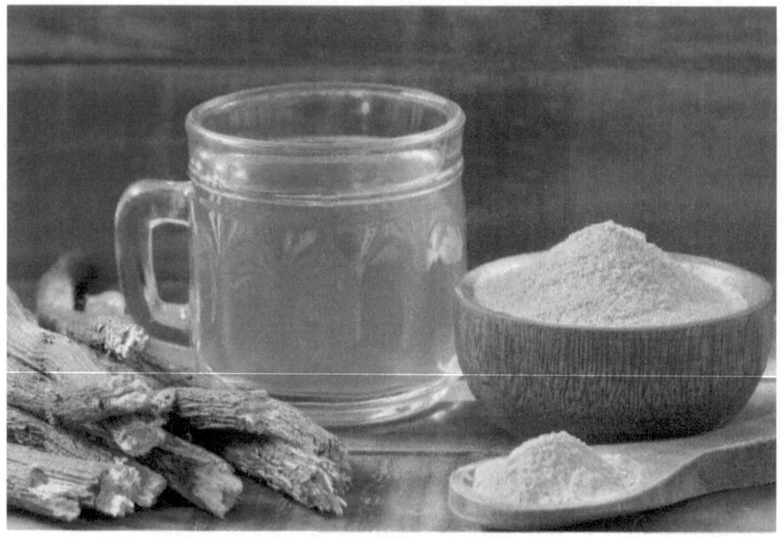

Here is a soother for your digestive system.

Serves: 2

Time: 25 mins.

Ingredients:

- ½ cup cinnamon chips
- 1 cup licorice root, dry & chopped
- ½ cup chamomile flowers
- 2 tablespoons whole cloves
- ½ cup orange peel, dried

Directions:

1. Mix everything together in a medium bowl & store the mixture in a glass jar in a cool place.

2. Now, over moderate heat in a large saucepan; mix 2 ½ cups of cold water with 3 heaping tablespoons of the mixture.

3. Bring everything to a boil. Once boiling, decrease the heat to low & simmer for 8 to 10 minutes.

4. Pour the tea into a large teacup using a strainer. Serve & enjoy!

Delicious Cherry Smoothie

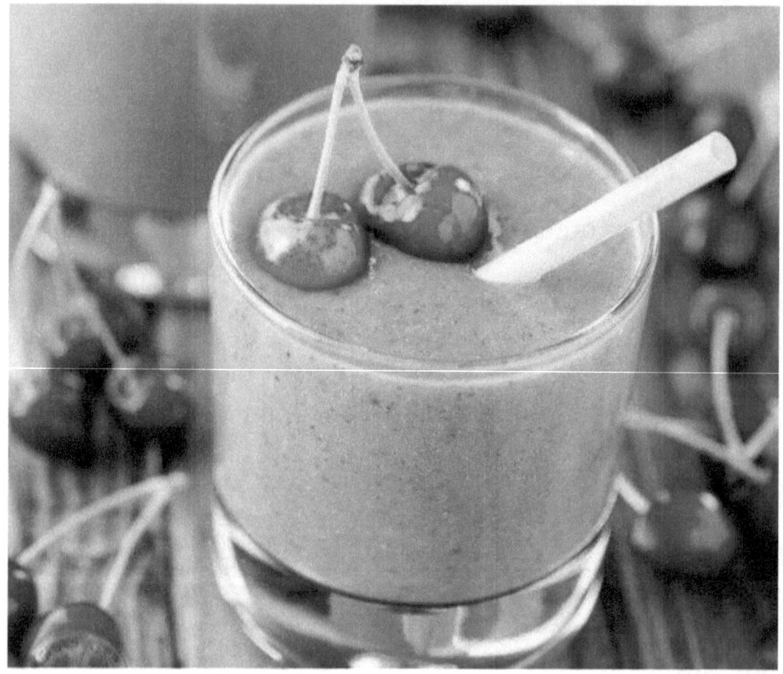

This combination of banana, frozen cherries, strawberries and almond milk are blende to make a satisfying drink.

Serves: 1

Time: 10 mins.

Ingredients:

- 1 banana, medium & organic
- 1 cup fresh or frozen cherries, organic, tart, pitted
- 1 ½ cups almond milk
- 1 cup strawberries, fresh & organic

Directions:

1. Put everything together in your blender & blend on high settings for a minute or two, until smooth.

2. Transfer the mixture in a large glass. Serve & enjoy.

Carrot Pineapple Smoothie

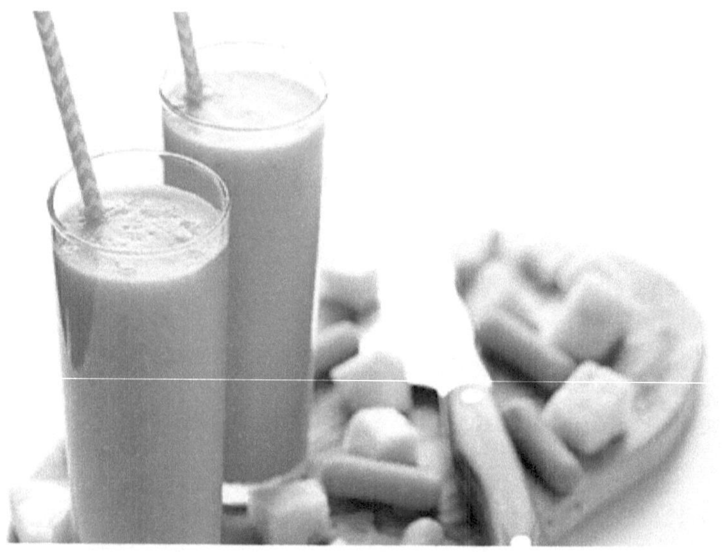

This no sugar added smoothie makes a bright and nutritious treat.

Serves: 2

Time: 10 mins.

Ingredients:

- 1 orange, peeled & deseeded
- 2 handfuls of baby spinach, fresh
- 1 & ½ cup pineapple, cubed
- 2 tablespoons chia seeds
- 1 carrot, large & chopped
- 8 ounces water
- ½ teaspoon ginger, fresh

Directions:

1. Put everything together in a blender & blend on high settings for a minute or two, until smooth.

2. Transfer the mixture into two large glasses. Serve & enjoy.

Kale Kiwi Smoothie

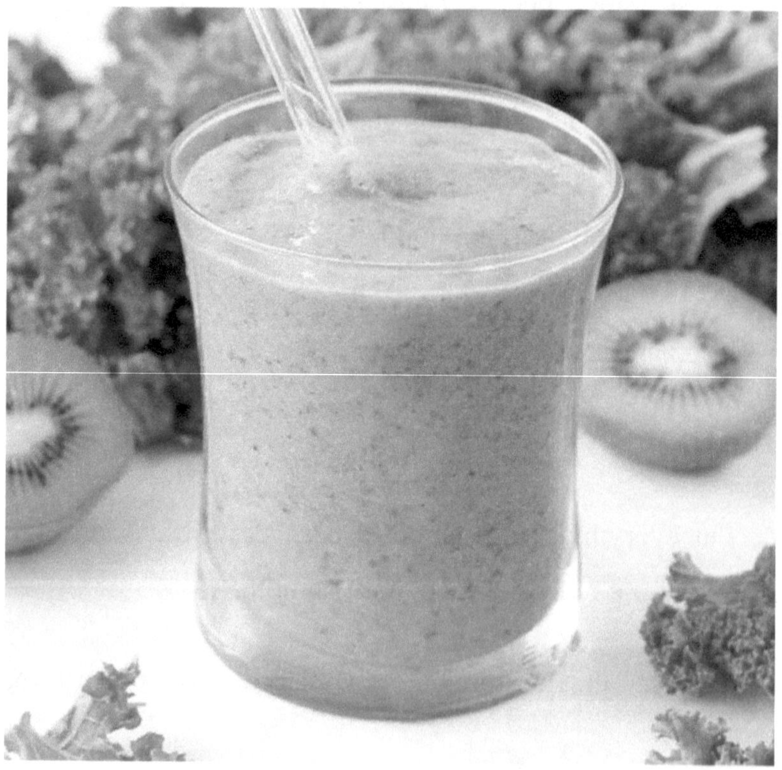

This Kale Kiwi Smoothie is surprisingly delicious and very good for you!

Serves: 2

Time: 15 mins.

Ingredients:

- 2 kiwifruits, peeled
- 1 mango, peeled & pitted
- 2 cups kale, torn or chopped
- 6 ounces filtered water

Directions:

1. Put everything together in a blender & blend on high settings for a minute or two, until smooth.

2. Transfer the mixture into two large glasses. Serve & enjoy.

Tart Cherry Lemonade

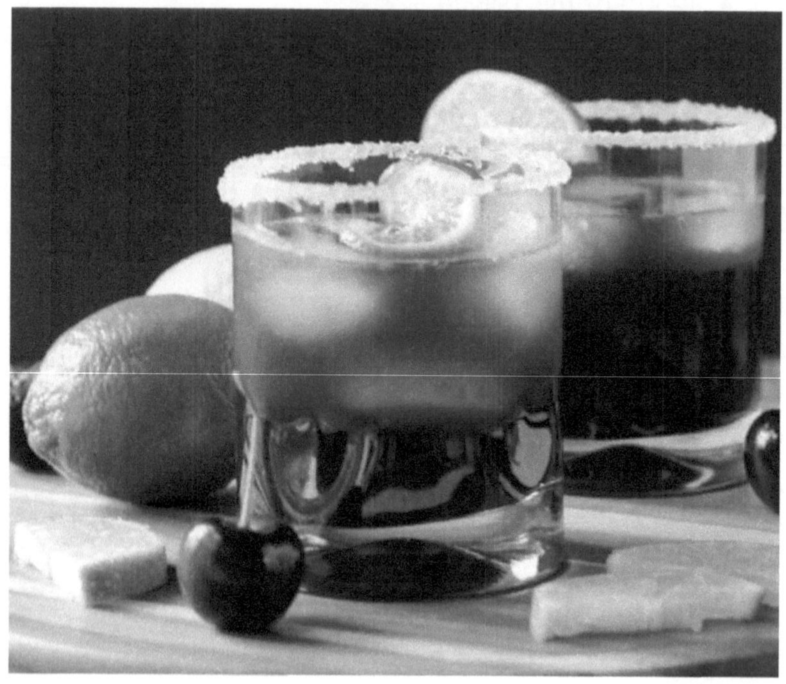

Sweet, a little fizzy and tart. Very easy to make and is fit for a perfect Summer sip.

Serves: 2

Time: 7 mins.

Ingredients:

- ¾ cup lemon juice, freshly squeezed
- 3 cups sparkling water or club soda
- 2 cups pure tart cherry juice, unsweetened
- Sweetener & ice cubes

Directions:

1. Transfer everything together in a large bowl; mix well.

2. To sweeten your drink, feel free to add sweetener to taste, if desired

3. Transfer the mix into two large chilled glasses; add in some ice cubes. Serve immediately & enjoy.

Orange Strawberry Smoothie

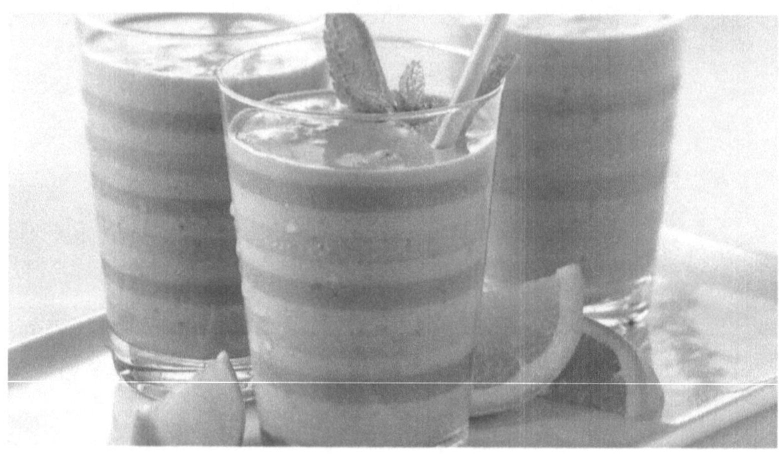

A refreshing icy, smooth blend of strawberries, baby spinach, orange and banana.

Serves: 4

Time: 25 mins.

Ingredients:

- 4 whole strawberries, large
- 2 handfuls baby spinach, fresh
- 1 orange, deseeded
- 6 ounces filtered water
- 1 banana, large, peeled & sliced

Directions:

1. Put everything together in a blender. Blend on high settings for a minute or two until smooth.

2. Transfer the mixture into two large chilled glasses. Serve & enjoy!

Mango Melon Delight

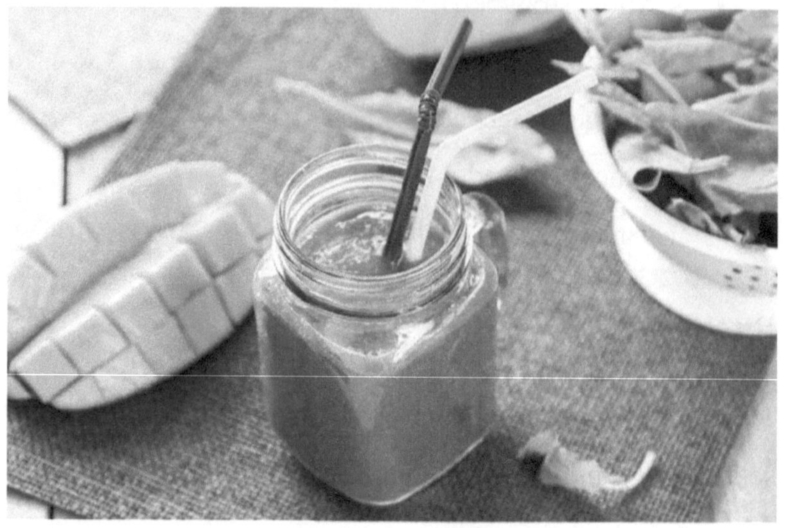

This refreshing drink is always a delight on those hot summer days.

Serves: 2

Time: 10 mins.

Ingredients:

- 4 strawberries, medium
- 1 cup cantaloupe, cubed
- 2 handfuls baby spinach, fresh
- 1 mango, peeled & pitted
- 4 to 6 ounces filtered water

Directions:

1. Put everything together in a blender. Blend on high settings for a minute or two until completely smooth.

2. Transfer the mixture into two large chilled glasses. Serve & enjoy!

Pineapple Grapefruit Smoothie

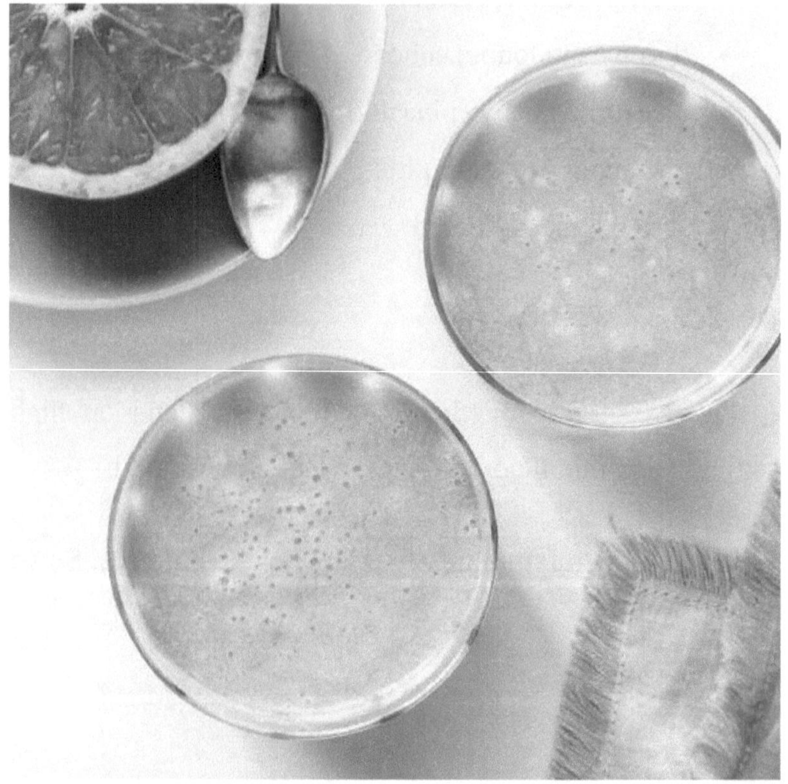

A perfect smoothie for dieting and it will always brighten your day.

Serves: 2

Time: 10 mins.

Ingredients:

- ½ cucumber, with peel
- 1 banana, fresh or frozen, peeled & sliced
- ½ cup pineapple, cubed
- 2 handfuls baby spinach, fresh or ½ cup parsley, fresh
- ½ red grapefruit, peeled
- 4 to 6 ounces filtered water

Directions:

1. Put everything together in a blender & blend on high settings for a minute or two, until smooth.

2. Transfer the mixture into two large glasses. Serve & enjoy.

Goat Cheese & Eggplant Sandwiches

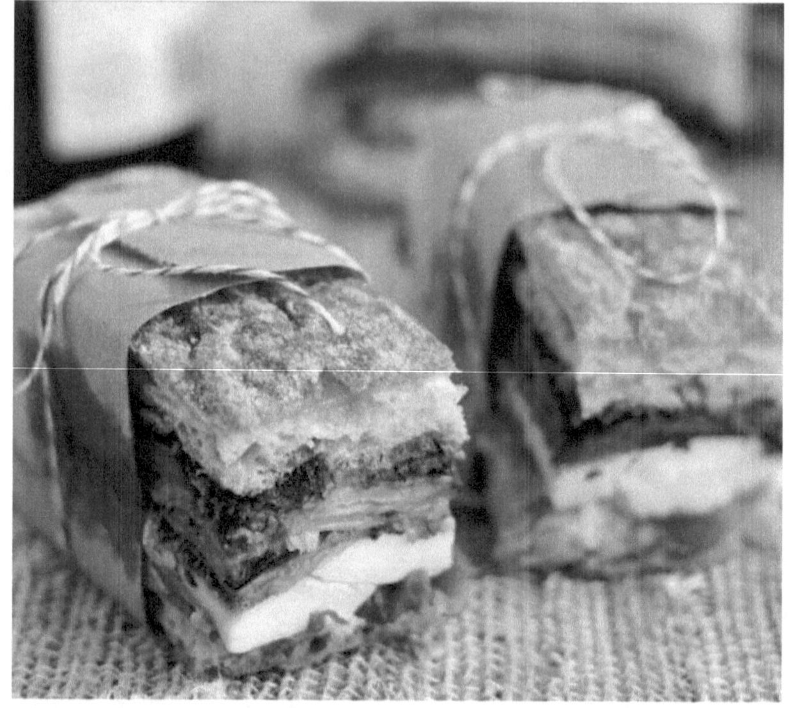

This is a hearty vegetable laden stacker. Transform sandwich night with this nutritious sandwich.

Serves: 2

Time: 30 mins.

Ingredients:

- 1 cup arugula
- 2 tomato slices (¼")
- ¼ cup goat cheese, softened (2 ounces)
- 2 eggplant, small, ¼" vertical slices
- ¼ teaspoon freshly ground black pepper
- 2 rustic sandwich rolls (1 ½ ounce)
- ¼ teaspoon salt
- 1 teaspoon olive oil

Directions:

1. Preheat your oven to 275 F in advance.

2. Lightly brush the eggplant with oil.

3. Lightly coat your large nonstick skillet with the cooking spray & heat it over medium-high heat.

4. Now, cook the eggplant until lightly browned, around 5 minutes per side. Sprinkle with pepper & salt.

5. Spread approximately a tablespoon of the goat cheese over each roll half, cut side.

6. Place the cheese sides of the rolls up on a large baking sheet; bake in the preheated oven until thoroughly heated, for 8 to 10 minutes.

7. Remove from your oven; top bottom half of every roll with ½ cup arugula, 1. Top your sandwiches with top halves of slice of tomato & 1 slice of eggplant the rolls.

Tomato Crostini

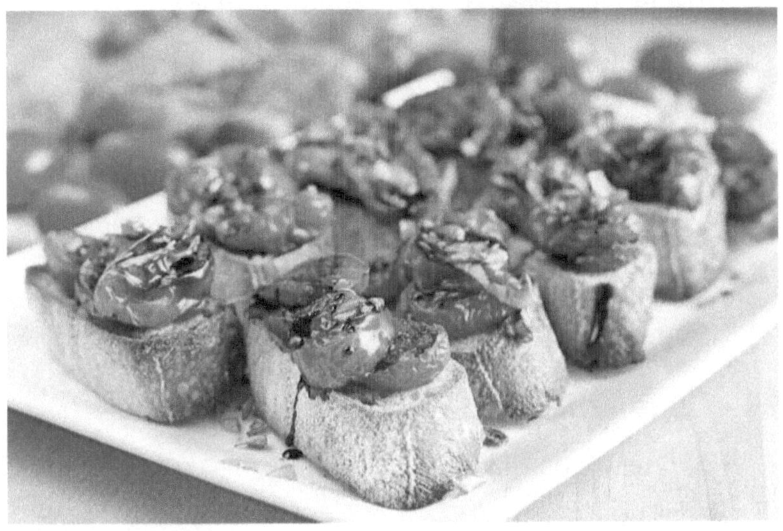

This is a fresh, tasty, flavorful dish. Just right for your special summer gatherings with friends.

Serves: 2

Time: 30 mins.

Ingredients:

- 4 French bread baguette slices (1" thick)
- 1 tablespoon green olives, chopped, pitted
- ½ cup plum tomato, chopped
- 1 teaspoon capers
- ½ teaspoon balsamic vinegar
- 1 tablespoon basil, fresh, chopped
- ⅛ teaspoon sea salt
- 1 clove garlic, halved
- ½ teaspoon olive oil
- 1 clove garlic, minced
- A dash of black pepper, freshly ground

Directions:

1. Preheat your oven to 375 F in advance.

2. Combine everything together (except the baguette & garlic clove halved) in a large bowl.

3. Lightly coat the slices of bread, both sides with the cooking spray & then arrange them on a large baking sheet in a single layer.

4. Bake in the preheated oven until lightly toasted, for 4 minutes per side.

5. Rub the halved garlic on one side of the bread slices & then evenly top with the tomato mixture.

Zesty Zucchini Spaghetti

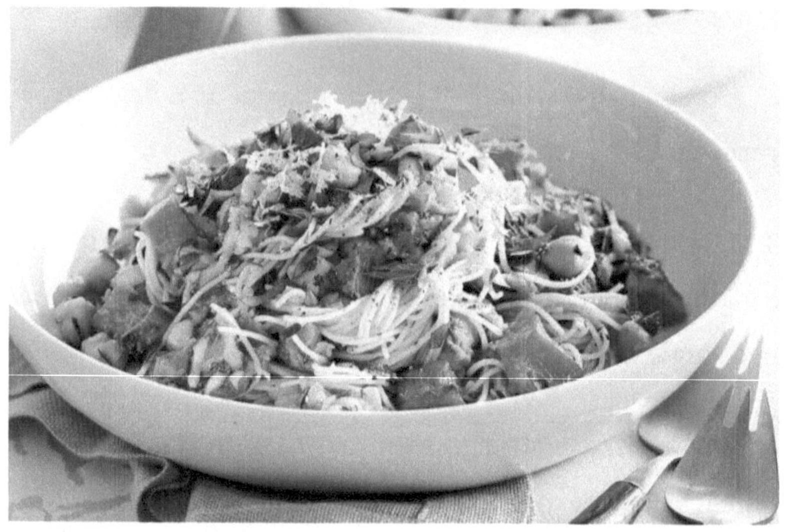

Spicy, rich in flavor and delicious. You are sure to enjoy.

Serves: 4

Time: 35 mins.

Ingredients:

- 1 & ¼ pounds zucchini, shredded (approximately 4 cups)
- 2 cloves garlic, minced
- ¾ pound uncooked spaghetti
- 2 tablespoons Parmesan cheese, shaved
- ¼ teaspoon black pepper
- 1 can of chipotle chilies in adobo sauce (7-ounce)
- 2 teaspoons olive oil
- ¾ teaspoon salt

Directions:

1. Cook the pasta as per the directions provided by the manufacturer; omit fat & salt.

2. Remove 1 tablespoon of sauce & 1 chili from the can. Remove the chili seeds and then mince the chili. Over medium-high heat in a non-stick large skillet; heat the oil.

3. Add in the sauce, chili & garlic; sauté for a minute and then add in the zucchini; cook for couple of minutes, stirring constantly.

4. Toss the prepared pasta with the zucchini mixture. Sprinkle with pepper, salt & cheese.

Rosemary-Roasted Potatoes

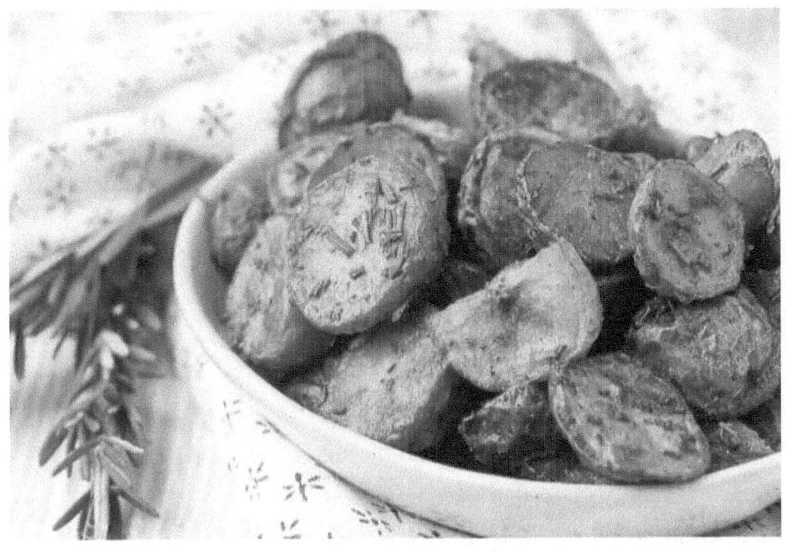

Here is a very flexible, easy and delicious side dish.

Serves: 4

Time: 30 mins.

Ingredients:

- 1 package red potato wedges, refrigerated (1-pound, 4-ounce)
- 2 tablespoons rosemary, fresh & chopped
- ½ teaspoon onion powder
- 1 tablespoon olive oil
- 3 cloves garlic, crushed
- ¼ teaspoon each salt & pepper

Directions:

1. Preheat your oven to 500 F in advance.

2. Combine everything together in a large bowl, mix well.

3. Thoroughly toss until each potato wedge is evenly coated with the seasonings & oil.

4. Line a large baking sheet with a foil & arrange the potato wedges it.

5. Bake in the preheated oven until tender and golden, for 20 to 22 minutes. Serve hot & enjoy.

Peaches with Berry Sauce

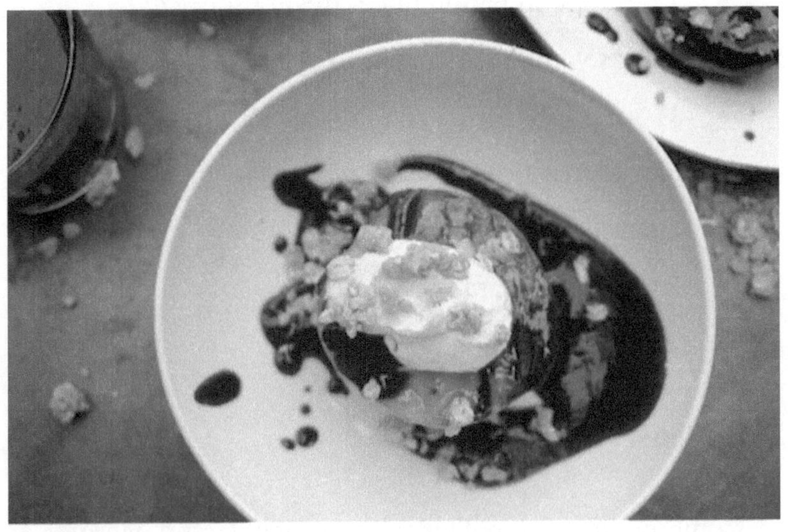

Very unusual dessert but it is pretty and delicious.

Serves: 4

Time: 20 mins.

Ingredients:

- 1 tablespoon lemon juice, freshly squeezed
- 2 cups vanilla ice cream, low-fat
- 1 cup berries, fresh such as raspberries, blackberries, strawberries
- 2 peaches, pitted & sliced
- 1 tablespoon Grand Marnier
- 2 tablespoons honey

Directions:

1. Combine honey together with berries, Grand Marnier & lemon juice in a blender.

2. Blend on high settings until smooth, for a minute. Using a fine sieve; strain into a bowl; discarding the seeds, if any & set aside.

3. Place a slice of peach in four dessert bowls & add ½ cup of the ice cream to every bowl; drizzle with the prepared berry sauce. Serve & enjoy!

Mini Raspberry Tarts

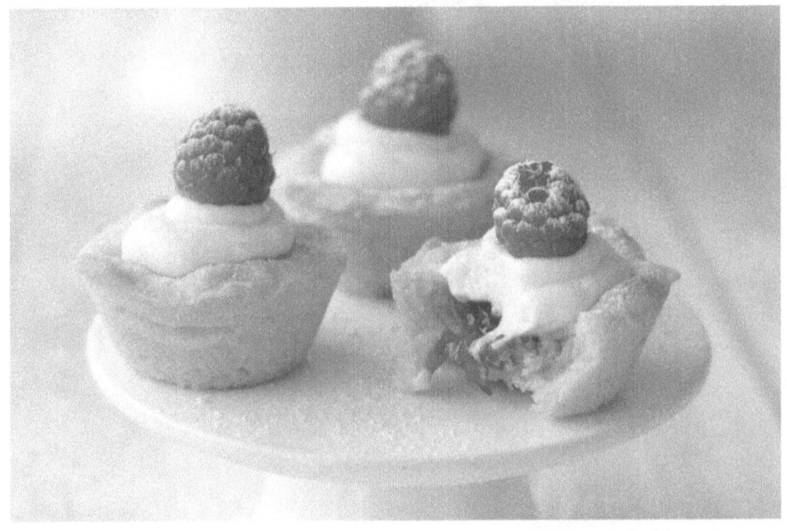

Perfect afternoon tea-time treats and great for picnics too.

Serves: 32

Time: 40 mins.

Ingredients:

- 32 raspberries, fresh
- 1 package of refrigerated sugar cookie dough (16.5-ounce)
- ¼ cup sugar
- 1 package cream cheese, block-style (8-ounce)
- ½ teaspoon vanilla extract
- Zest of 1 orange, fresh

Directions:

1. Preheat your oven to 350 F in advance.

2. Using nonstick cooking spray; lightly coat a mini-muffin tin.

3. Evenly divide the cookie dough into 32 pieces. Coat the pieces in flour & roll into balls using your hands.

4. Press every ball into the tin, forming dough up. Bake until golden, for 10 to 12 minutes.

5. Once done, let them cool for couple of minutes in the pan. Remove the tarts & transfer them on a wire rack to completely cool.

6. Now, combine sugar together with cream cheese, vanilla & orange zest using an electric mixer in a large bowl. Spoon the cream cheese mixture into every tart. Top all of the 32 tarts with a fresh raspberry. Place in a refrigerator & let chill until ready to use. Serve & enjoy.

Pumpkin Pancakes

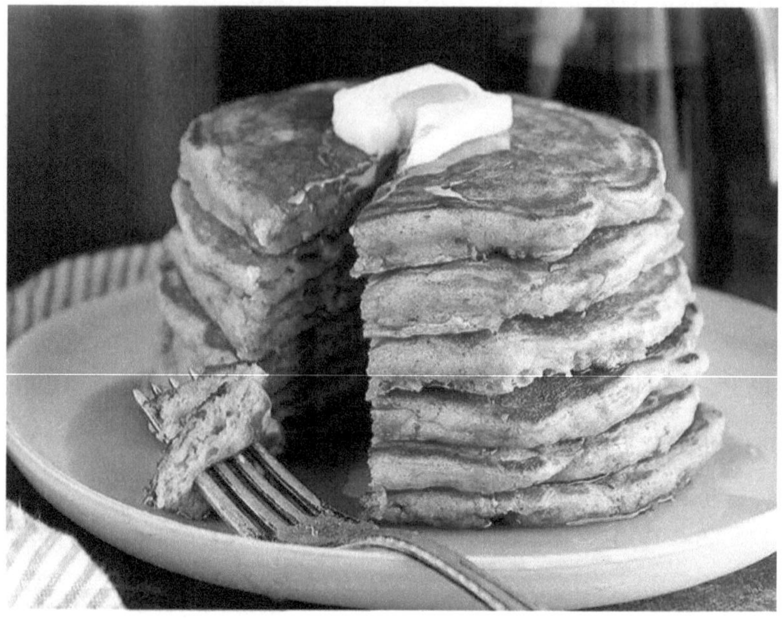

This pumpkin recipe will become your favorite. Fluffy and nutritious.

Serves: 4

Time: 10 mins.

Ingredients:

- ¼ teaspoon baking soda
- 4 egg whites, large
- ¼ cup cake flour
- 1 egg yolk, large
- ½ cup vanilla yogurt, low-fat
- Cooking spray
- ¼ teaspoon salt
- Honey or Maple syrup
- ½ cup pumpkin, canned

Directions:

1. Whisk pumpkin together with egg yolk, baking soda, flour, and yogurt in a large bowl.

2. Whisk the egg whites with salt & then fold the mixture into the bowl with the pumpkin mixture.

3. Lightly coat a large nonstick skillet with the cooking spray & heat over medium heat.

For each pancake:

4. Pour down 1/3 cup of the batter into the hot skillet & cook for 2 to 3 minutes.

5. When the edges are slightly brown, and you can see the bubbles on the tops; flip & cook the other side for couple of more minutes. Drizzle honey or maple syrup over the top.

Cornflakes, Berries & Low-Fat Milk

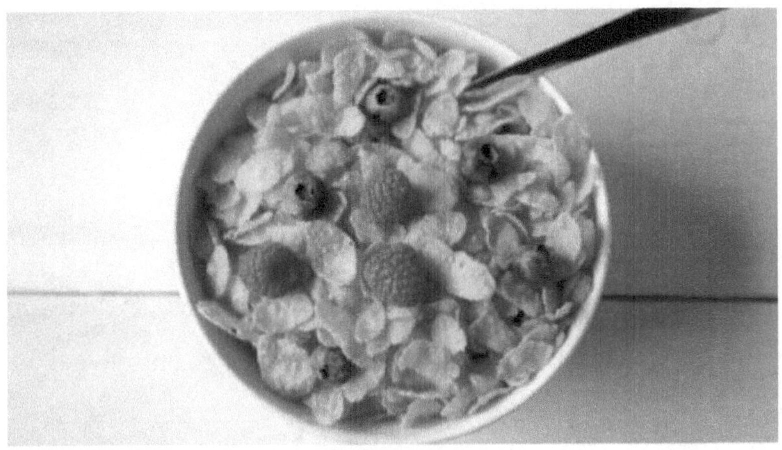

A great start to your day. Very colorful and nutritious.

Serves: 2

Time: 7 mins.

Ingredients:

- 1 cup berries, fresh
- 2 cups cornflakes
- 1 cup milk, 1% low-fat

Directions:

1. Place the cornflakes in a small sized bowl & then top your bowl with milk & fresh berries. Serve & enjoy!

Savory Cabbage Pancakes

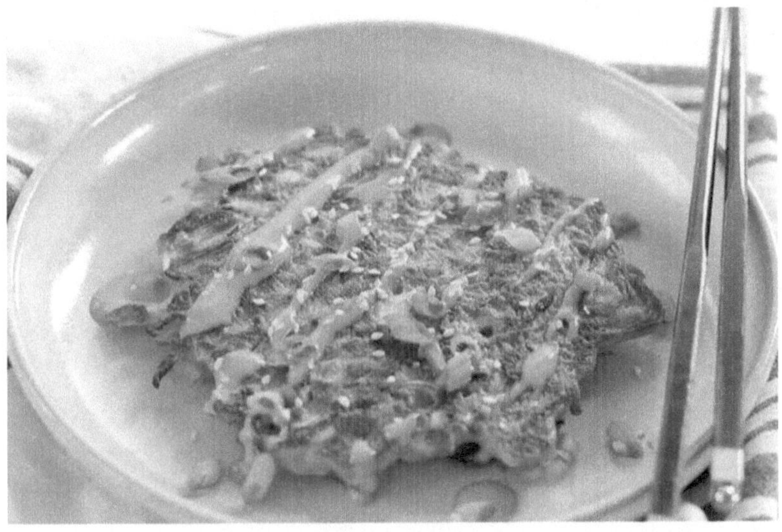

Mouthwatering, you are certainly in for a treat if you have never tasted these cabbage pancakes before.

Serves: 6

Time: 30 mins.

Ingredients:

For Pancakes:

- 5 cups green cabbage, remove any wilted leaves, cut into quarters, remove the core & thinly sliced or shredded
- ¾ to 1 cup flour, all-purpose
- 2 eggs, extra-large
- 1 tablespoon sesame oil, toasted
- 3 green onions, sliced
- 1 ½ tablespoon soy sauce
- 1 carrot, medium, peeled & shredded using a cheese grater
- ½ cup water
- 2 tablespoons oil

For Toppings:

- ½ tablespoon sesame seeds
- 2 green onions
- ¼ cup mayonnaise
- 2 tablespoons Sriracha

Directions:

1. Whisk the eggs together with water, sesame oil & soy sauce until smooth in a large bowl.

2. Start with whisking ¼ cup of the flour, until it forms a smooth & thick batter.

3. Add in the green onion, cabbage & carrots to the batter; give everything a good stir until the vegetables are evenly mixed & coated with the batter.

4. Over medium heat in a cast iron or non-stick skillet; heat approximately half tablespoon of oil.

5. Once hot, add ¾ cup of vegetable & batter mixture; pressing it down into the hot skillet & make a circle (approximately ½" thick & 6" in diameter).

6. Cover & cook the pancake for couple of minutes, until the bottom turns golden brown; flip & cook the other side for couple of more minutes, until golden brown as well.

7. Mound the cooked pancakes on a large plate; cover with an aluminum foil until ready to eat.

8. As you cook the pancakes, feel free to add more of oil to the skillet, if required.

For Sriracha mayo:

9. Combine ¼ cup of mayonnaise together with 2 tablespoons of Sriracha in a small bowl.

10. Just before serving, drizzle the Sriracha mayo on top of the cooked pancakes followed with a sprinkle of sliced green onion & sesame seeds.

Carrot Cake Pancakes

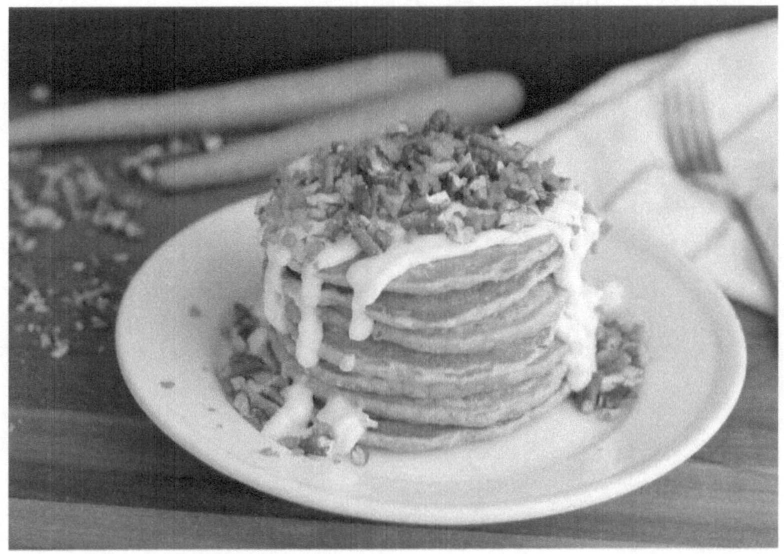

Wow, these are some tasty pancakes! Fluffy, packed with aromatic spices and slightly sweet.

Serves: 8

Time: 40 mins.

Ingredients:

- ½ teaspoon cloves, ground
- 2 cups complete pancake mix
- ½ cup brown sugar, packed
- ⅓ cup raisins, packed
- ¾ cup carrots, raw & shredded
- 2 teaspoons cinnamon, ground
- ½ teaspoon nutmeg, ground
- A dash of salt
- 1 ½ cups water

Directions:

1. Combine pancake mix with water in a large bowl; mix well.

2. Combine the leftover ingredients in a separate bowl.

3. Gently fold the carrot mixture into the pancake batter; let rest for couple of minutes at room temperature.

4. Pour approximately ¼ cup of the batter onto a griddle, lightly greased.

5. Cook for couple of minutes until slightly golden brown; flip and cook the other side as well.

Overnight Oats with Flax & Cinnamon

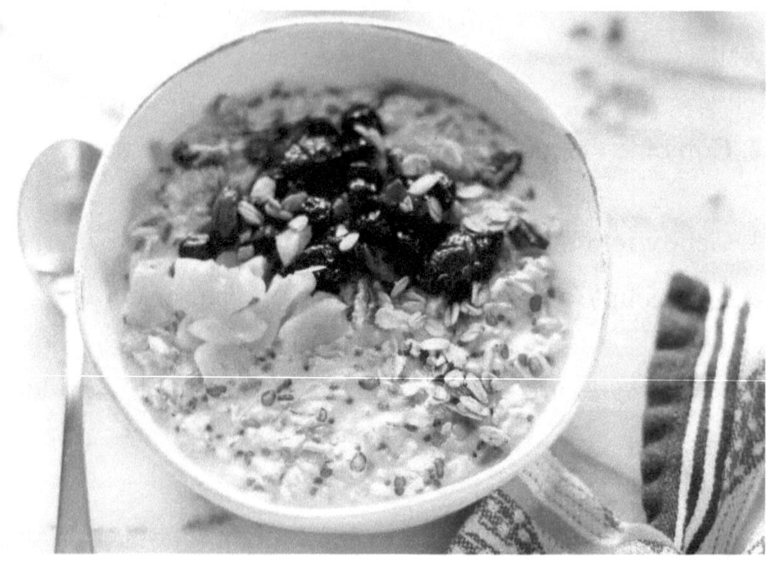

This is a healthy start to your morning. Very satisfying and energizing.

Serves: 2

Time: 25 mins.

Ingredients:

- 4 cups almond milk, unsweetened
- 1 teaspoon maple syrup
- 2 cups rolled oats, gluten-free
- ⅛ teaspoon sea salt
- 2 tablespoons ground flax seeds
- 1 teaspoon cinnamon

Directions:

1. Combine everything together in a large glass bowl; give everything a good stir. Cover & let refrigerate for overnight.

2. The next morning; mix a cup of overnight refrigerated oats with approximately 1 tablespoon of flax seeds & ¼ teaspoon of cinnamon.

3. Drizzle with a splash of more milk and a teaspoon of maple syrup. Serve & enjoy!

Creamy Chocolate Avocado Ice Cream

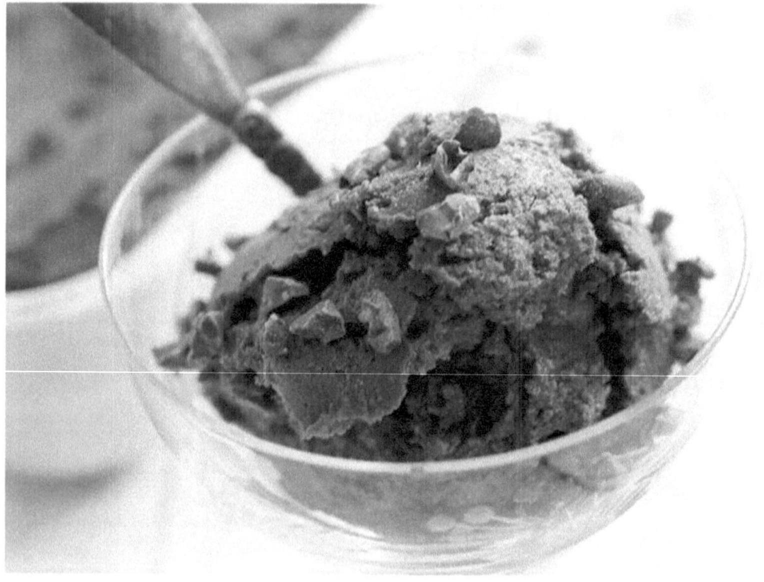

This refreshing ice cream is so creamy and incredibly delicious!

Serves: 1

Time: 4 hrs. 5 mins.

Ingredients:

- 1 can coconut milk, full fat (13.5 ounce)
- ½ cup plus 2 tablespoons maple syrup
- 1 avocado, peeled & pitted
- Hot fudge (Vegan, for drizzling)
- ½ cup cocoa powder, unsweetened
- 1 tablespoon vanilla extract
- ½ cup water
- sprinkles (Vegan, for sprinkling on top)

Directions:

1. Add coconut milk & avocado to a blender or food processor & pulse on high settings until smooth.

2. Add in the leftover ingredients & blend on high settings again until smooth & well incorporated, for 2 minutes, scraping down the bowl once.

3. Place all the base of your ice cream into a freezer safe container & then place the container in a freezer; let freeze for a minimum period of an hour to 4 hours.

4. After every 20 minutes, whisk slightly.

5. When ready to eat; add hot fudge and sprinkles on top & scoop out using an ice cream scoop.

Vanilla Bean Pudding

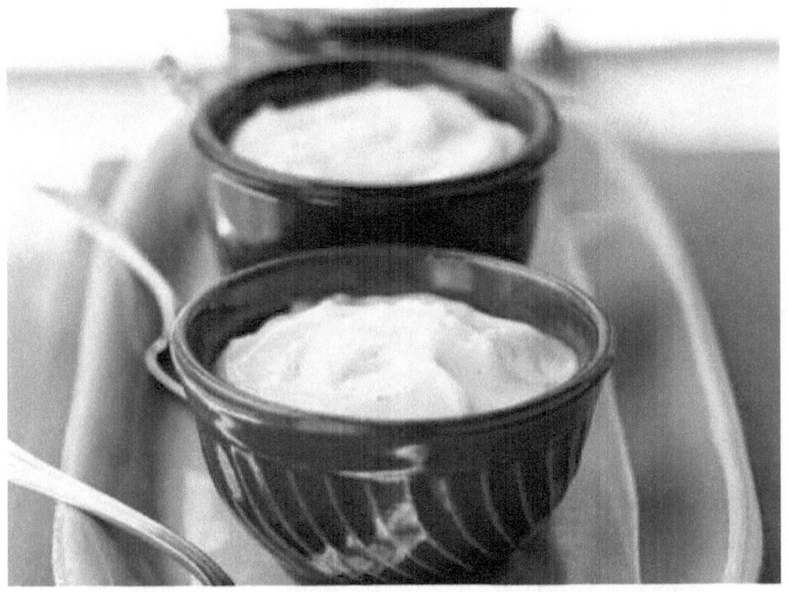

Nothing better than a good old-fashioned homemade ice cream made from scratch.

Serves: 6

Time: 30 mins.

Ingredients:

- 3 tablespoons cornstarch
- 1 vanilla bean, split lengthwise
- 4 teaspoons butter
- ¼ cup half-and-half
- 2 ½ cups milk, 2% reduced fat
- ¾ cup sugar
- 2 egg yolks, large
- ⅛ teaspoon salt

Directions:

1. Scrape the seeds from vanilla bean. Pour milk together with the bean and seeds in a medium, heavy saucepan. Bring to a boil over moderate heat.

2. Now, in a large bowl; combine cornstarch together with sugar & salt; give everything a good stir.

3. Combine egg yolks with half & half, stir well. Stir the egg yolk mixture into the sugar mixture.

4. Slowly add ½ of hot milk into the sugar mixture, continue to stir with a whisk.

5. Put the hot milk mixture to the pan again; bring to a boil & cook for a minute, continue to stir with a whisk.

6. Remove the pan from heat. Add in the butter, continue to stir until butter melts completely.

7. Remove & discard the vanilla bean. Spoon the pudding into a medium bowl.

8. Place the pudding bowl in a large bowl filled with the ice until the pudding cools, for 15 minutes, stirring occasionally. Cover the surface using a plastic wrap & let chill.

Banana Nut Bread

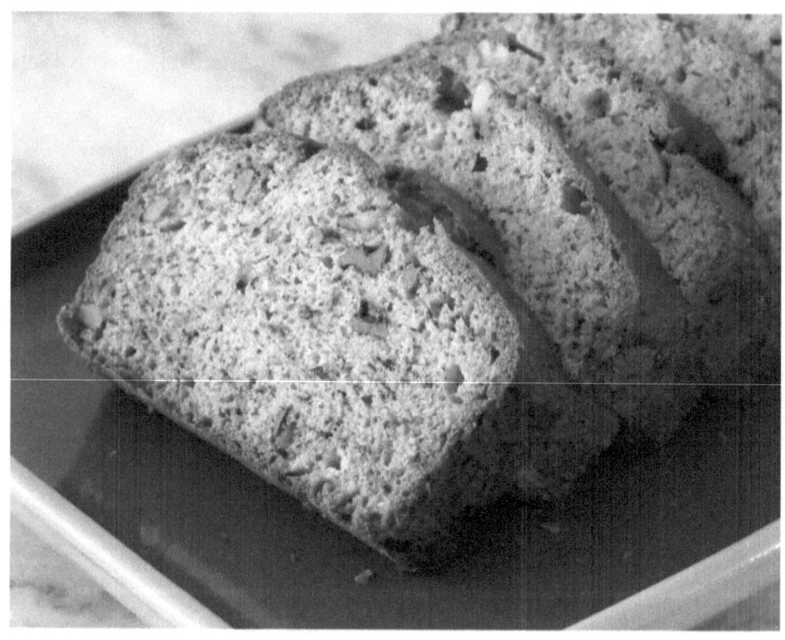

This delicious Banana Nut Bread is moist, sweet and flavorful!

Serves: 8

Time: 1 hr. 40 mins.

Ingredients:

- ½ cup pecans, chopped coarsely
- 1 egg yolk, large
- ¼ cup wheat germ
- 1 teaspoon canola oil
- ⅔ cup Splenda or stevia
- ½ teaspoon pure vanilla extract
- 2 bananas, medium
- ¼ cup buttermilk, low-fat
- 3 egg whites, large
- ½ teaspoon cinnamon, ground
- 1 ¼ cup all-purpose white flour
- ¾ cup whole wheat flour
- 2 teaspoons baking powder
- ¼ teaspoon nutmeg, ground
- 2 teaspoons light brown sugar
- ½ teaspoon baking soda
- ¼ teaspoon salt

Directions:

1. Preheat the oven to 350 F in advance. Line a glass loaf pan, 1 ½ quart with non-stick foil.

2. Whisk the egg yolk for couple of minutes, until smooth. Add in the canola oil; whisk until completely smooth.

3. Mash the bananas into the mixture using the whisk until smooth. Add in the vanilla extract & Splenda; whisk until smooth, for couple of minutes.

4. Whisk the egg whites in separate bowl until very white & frothy.

5. Place the whole-wheat flour together with all-purpose flour, baking soda, baking powder, cinnamon, salt, wheat germ & nutmeg in a sifter; sift into the mixing bowl.

6. Gently fold in the creamed mixture with flour mixture. As you blend add in the chopped pecans followed by the frothed egg whites & fold them together until smooth.

7. Add in the buttermilk & fold again until smooth.

8. Transfer the batter into the lined loaf pan dish & evenly sprinkle the brown sugar on the top.

9. Place the loaf pan into your oven & bake until done, for 50 to 55 minutes.

Avocado Chocolate Bread

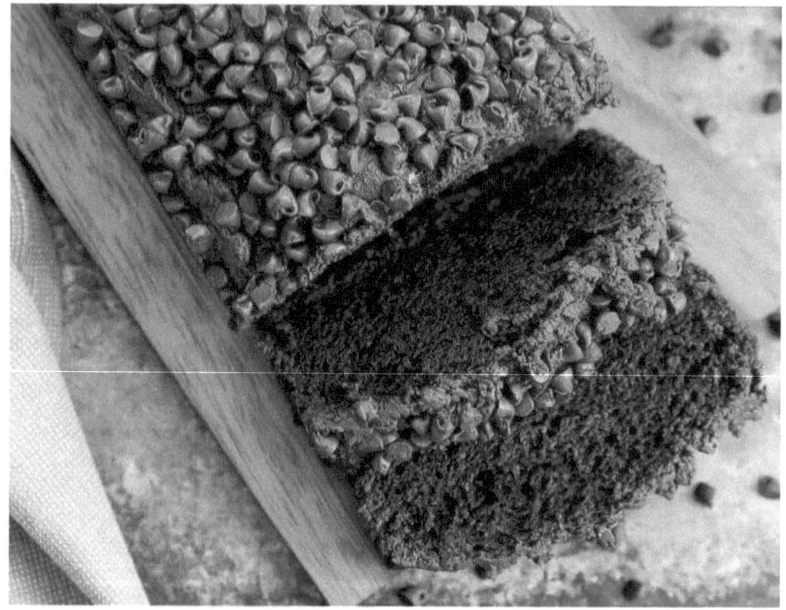

This supremely decadent Avocado Chocolate Bread is healthy, super moist and mouthwatering.

Serves: 8

Time: 1 hr. 30 mins.

Ingredients:

- 3 tablespoons honey, raw
- 1 ½ cups avocado
- 3 tablespoons coconut oil, melted
- 1 teaspoon vanilla extract
- 2 eggs at room temperature
- ¼ cup cacao powder, raw
- 2 ½ tablespoons coconut cream
- ½ cup pecans
- 2 cups almond flour, blanched
- ⅓ cup plus some more chocolate chips
- 1 teaspoon baking soda
- ½ teaspoon salt

Directions:

1. Line the sides and bottom of a medium loaf pan, 8½ x 4½" with the parchment paper & preheat your oven to 350 F.

2. Add avocado to the food processor; pulse on high until you get the pieces.

3. Then add in the coconut cream, vanilla, coconut oil, eggs, and honey; pulse on high settings again until smooth.

4. Add the chopped pecans along with the cacao powder, baking soda, almond flour, chocolate chips and salt into a large bowl.

5. Gently mix the dry & wet ingredients together using a rubber spatula. Don't over mix.

6. Spoon the batter into the pan already prepared & sprinkle chocolate chips over the top.

7. Bake batter until toothpick inserted comes out clean, roughly 45 minutes.

8. Let cool in the pan over a wire rack for 10 minutes before serving.

Chicken & Barley Soup

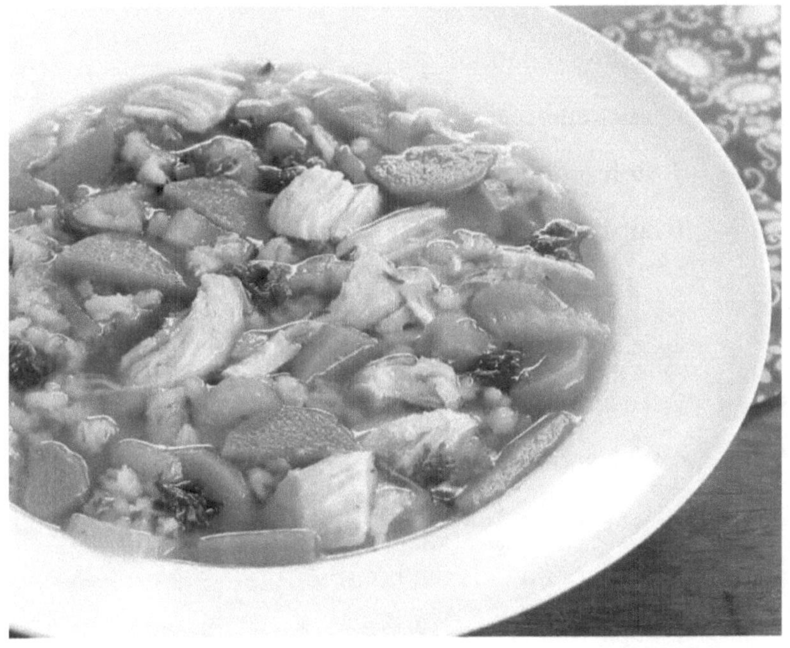

This is a very filling and hearty main dish. Your family will love it.

Serves: 10

Time: 1 hr.

Ingredients:

- 2 cups barley
- 1 yellow onion, diced
- 4 chicken breasts, boneless, skinless
- 1 tablespoon garlic, minced
- 6 cups chicken broth
- 2 - 3 carrots, large, chopped
- 1 celery stalk, chopped
- 2 teaspoons parsley, dried
- 1 tablespoon flour
- ½ teaspoon ground sage
- 1 tablespoon chicken bouillon
- 3 cups water
- 1 teaspoon thyme, dried
- Olive oil
- Pepper & salt to taste

Directions:

1. Over medium high heat in a large Dutch oven; heat 2 tablespoons of olive oil.

2. Once hot; sauté the onions together with carrots & celery for 3 to 4minutes, until softened.

3. Add in the minced garlic & sauté for a minute more. Add in the flour; give everything a good stir.

4. Pour in the chicken broth, 3 cups of water & bouillon. Add in the chicken breasts & barley; bring everything to a boil.

5. Once boiling, decrease the heat & let simmer for 20 minutes.

6. Carefully remove the chicken breasts using tongs; shred into small pieces & back to the pot again. Stir in thyme, parsley, sage, pepper & salt to taste.

7. Let simmer until barley is tender, for 15 to 20 more minutes. Serve & enjoy.

Arugula, Cherry & Quinoa Salad

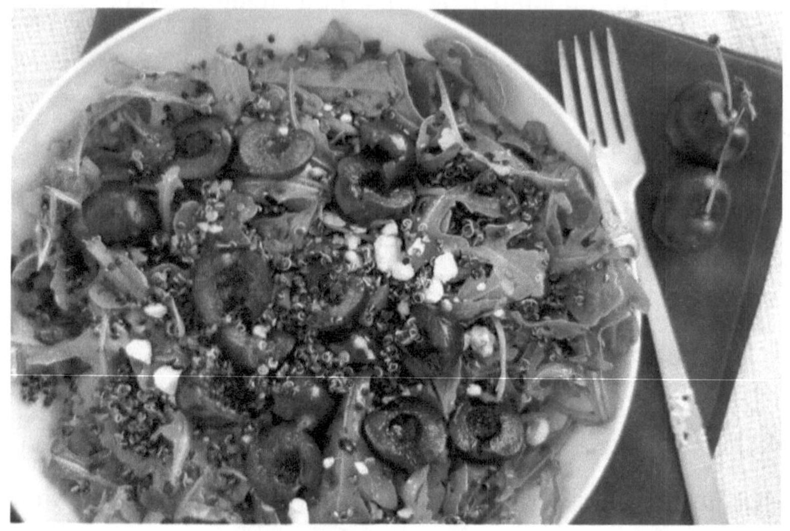

This salad is light, nutritious and incredibly simple to make.

Serves: 12

Time: 30 mins.

Ingredients:

For Dressing:

- 1 tablespoon olive oil
- 1 tablespoon balsamic vinegar
- 1 teaspoon Dijon mustard
- Pepper & salt to taste

For Salad:

- Goat cheese crumbles
- A handful of dark cherries, pitted & sliced in half
- Cooked quinoa (red or black), slightly warm
- Arugula, fresh

Directions:

1. In a suitable sized bowl, whisk all the dressing ingredients; toss with more than a few handfuls of Arugula.

2. Add in the quinoa & sprinkle with the goat cheese & cherries. Mix well. Serve & enjoy.

Quinoa Salad with Kale & Dark Cherries

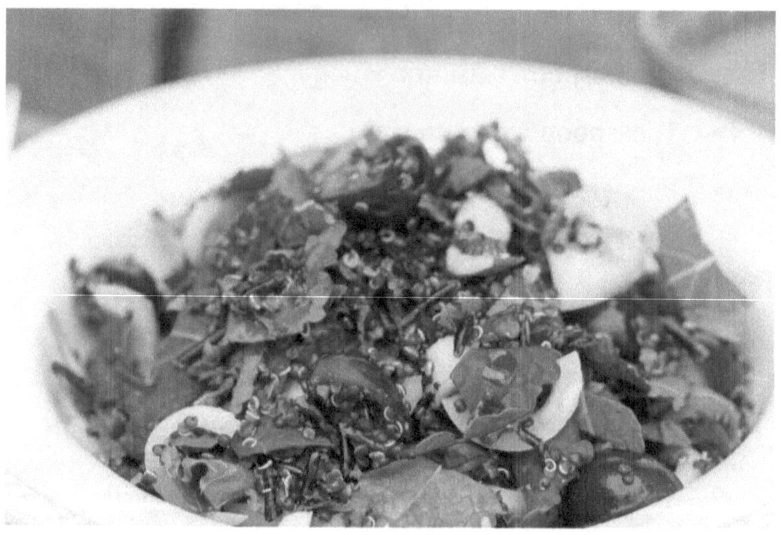

This refreshing salad is a delicious and healthy addition to any meal.

Serves: 4

Time: 50 mins.

Ingredients:

- 2 cups quinoa, cooked
- ½ cup nuts-almonds, chopped such as pecans or cashews; raw or sprouted
- ½ cup wild rice
- 1 cup kale, raw & chopped
- ½ cup celery, chopped
- 2 cups dark red cherries, pitted & halved
- ¼ cup olive oil, extra virgin
- Black pepper & sea salt to taste
- 1 garlic clove, minced
- ¼ cup apple cider vinegar
- 1 teaspoon Dijon mustard

Directions:

1. To remove the bitter coating; don't forget to soak the quinoa for a minimum period of 15 minutes and then drain

2. Cook the rice in 3 cups of water for 15 minutes, over high heat.

3. Now, add the drained quinoa to the cooked wild rice.

4. Continue cooking until al dente & just done, for 15 more minutes.

5. Drain the mixture & combine quinoa with the vegetables, wild rice mixture, nuts and cherries in a large sized bowl.

6. Whisk vinegar, together with oil, garlic, mustard, pepper & salt; pour this mixture on top of your salad.

Spicy Thai Chicken & Quinoa

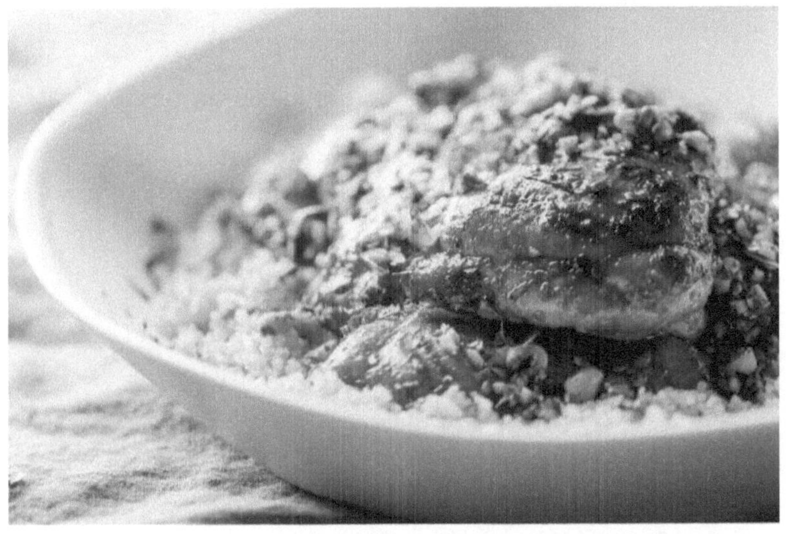

This sticky, delicious and saucy dish is a great main dish.

Serves: 4

Time: 50 mins.

Ingredients:

For the Chicken:

- 2 pounds chicken thighs, boneless, skinless
- Fresh cilantro, chili flakes & peanuts, chopped
- 2 cups quinoa, uncooked

For Spicy Thai Sauce:

- 2 tablespoons light brown sugar, organic
- ½ cup Thai style chili sauce
- 1 garlic clove, minced
- ½ cup chicken broth or water
- 2 tablespoons rice vinegar
- ¼ cup blue agave, organic
- 2 tablespoons lime juice
- ¼ cup soy sauce

Directions:

1. Whisk all the sauce and ingredients together in your large bowl; set approximately ½ cup of the sauce aside.

2. Bring the sauce to a boil over medium heat in a small saucepan.

3. Once boiling, decrease the heat to low & let simmer until the sauce has thickened, for half an hour.

4. In the meantime, keep cooking the quinoa as per the directions provided by the manufacturer.

5. Now, place the chicken in a bowl or bag with the kept ½ cup of the sauce & let marinate for half an hour in a refrigerator.

6. Shake off additional marinade & transfer the marinated pieces of chicken on a hot skillet or grill pan.

7. Keep cooking the chicken pieces until no longer pink, for couple of minutes on each side; don't forget to brush the chicken occasionally with the thickened sauce.

8. Place the cooked quinoa on a large platter & top it with the cooked pieces of chicken.

9. Brush everything completely with some more sauce. Sprinkle with peanuts, cilantro & the chili flakes.

Lemon & Sage Roasted Chicken

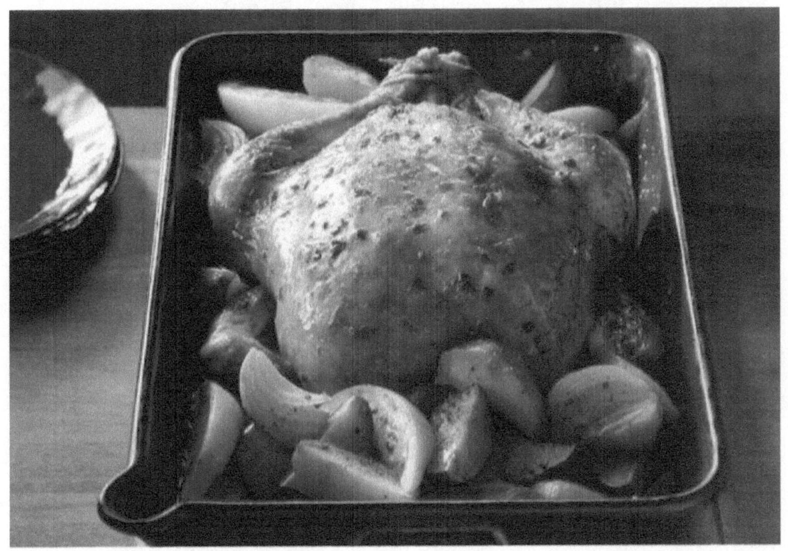

Simple roast chicken packed with flavor, goes well with fresh seasonal vegetable.

Serves: 4

Time: 2 hrs. 40mins.

Ingredients:

- ½ pound turnips, peeled & trimmed
- 2 lemons, sliced thinly
- 1 whole chicken (6 pound)
- 3 teaspoons olive oil, divided
- ¾ pound carrots, peeled & trimmed
- 6 sage leaves, fresh
- ¾ pound parsnips, peeled & trimmed
- 1 pound fingerling potatoes, halved
- 2 tablespoons thyme, fresh & chopped

Directions:

1. Preheat your oven to 425 F in advance. Place at least 6 slices of lemon & the sage leaves under the skin of your chicken.

2. Put the leftover lemon into the cavity. Tie the legs all together with the twine & tuck the wings under.

3. Brush all sides of the chicken with approximately 1 teaspoon of oil.

4. Place the chicken in your roasting pan & roast in the lower third of your oven until an instant thermometer reflects 165, for 1 hour 15 minutes.

5. Transfer the roasted chicken to a large cutting board & let rest for couple of minutes at room temperature.

6. In the meantime, cut the root vegetables into matchsticks. Toss with potatoes with thyme and leftover oil in a baking pan.

7. Roast until tender, for 45 minutes, stirring occasionally.

8. Remove the skin from chicken; discard the lemons slices from cavity & slice the cooked meat enough to serve. Serve the roasted chicken with half of the vegetables.

Basil Garlic Grilled Chicken Breasts

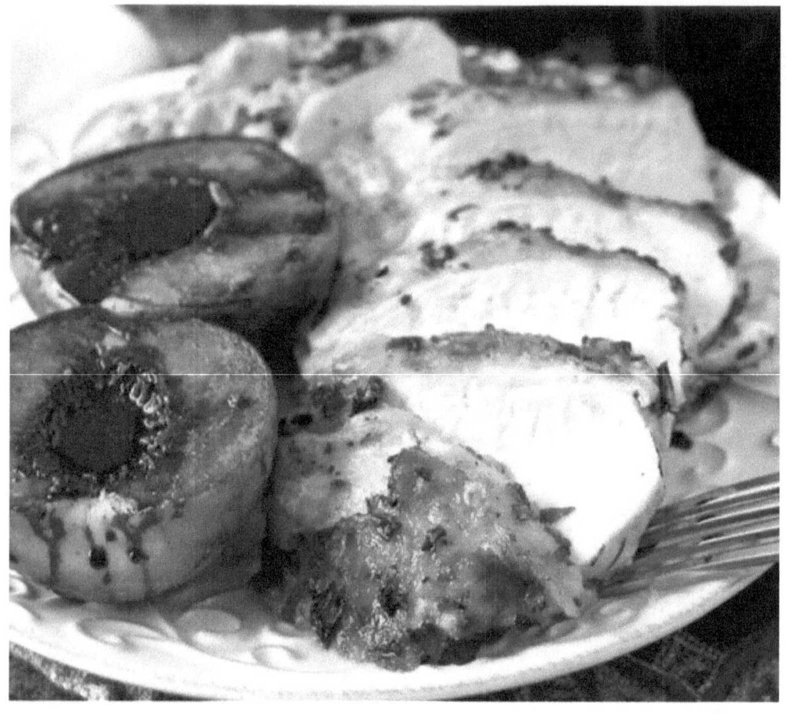

You will love the flavor of this grilled chicken breast. Makes a satisfying dinner for the entire family.

Serves: 4

Time: 1 hr.

Ingredients:

- 4 boneless chicken breast halves, large & skin-on (10 to 12 ounces each)
- ¼ cup extra virgin olive oil
- 3 tablespoons garlic, minced finely
- ½ cup basil, fresh & chopped
- Freshly ground black pepper & salt to taste

Directions:

1. Mix garlic together with oil & basil in a small bowl. If required, feel free to add more of oil.

2. Carefully smudge both sides of the chicken breasts with this mixture being; leaving the skins unbroken.

3. Sprinkle with pepper & salt; let marinate for couple of hours.

4. To crisp the skin; place the marinated chicken (skin side down) over a medium fire for 8 to 10 minutes.

5. Keep an eye on everything; ensure you don't burn the chicken.

6. Flip the chicken breasts over & cook the other side for 6 to 8 more minutes.

7. Remove from the heat & let rest for 10 minutes at room temperature. Serve & enjoy.

Conclusion

You did it! I'm elated that you stuck with us up to this point. Hopefully you have enjoyed. I hope you were able to prepare and enjoyed all 30 Brilliant Gout Recipes for A Hectic Lifestyle.

Please take some time to leave me a review on Amazon to let me know what you thought of the recipes.

Bye for now!

About the Author

Born in New Germantown, Pennsylvania, Stephanie Sharp received a Masters degree from Penn State in English Literature. Driven by her passion to create culinary masterpieces, she applied and was accepted to The International Culinary School of the Art Institute where she excelled in French cuisine. She has married her cooking skills with an aptitude for business by opening her own small cooking school where she teaches students of all ages.

Stephanie's talents extend to being an author as well and she has written over 400 e-books on the art of cooking and baking that include her most popular recipes.

Sharp has been fortunate enough to raise a family near her hometown in Pennsylvania where she, her husband and children live in a beautiful rustic house on an extensive piece of land. Her other passion is taking care of the furry members of her family which include 3 cats, 2 dogs and a potbelly pig named Wilbur.

Watch for more amazing books by Stephanie Sharp coming out in the next few months.

Author's Afterthoughts

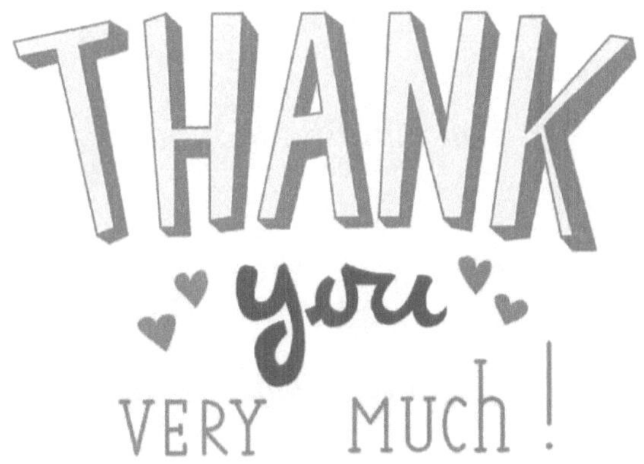

I am truly grateful to you for taking the time to read my book. I cherish all of my readers! Thanks ever so much to each of my cherished readers for investing the time to read this book!

With so many options available to you, your choice to buy my book is an honour, so my heartfelt thanks at reading it from beginning to end!

I value your feedback, so please take a moment to submit an honest and open review on Amazon so I can get valuable insight into my readers' opinions and others can benefit from your experience.

Thank you for taking the time to review!

Stephanie Sharp

For announcements about new releases, please follow my author page on Amazon.com!

You can find that at:

https://www.amazon.com/author/stephanie-sharp

*or Scan **QR-code** below.*